The Preventive Vet's **Start Off On The Right Paw**™ Series

101 Essential Tips

You Need to Raise a Happy, Healthy, Safe Dog

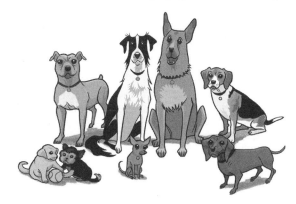

Jason Nicholas, BVetMed

Illustrated by Chuck Gonzales

The Preventive Vet
Portland, Oregon

ISBN: 978-0-9883781-1-7

Book cover and interior design by Anita Jones, Another Jones Graphics
Illustrations by Chuck Gonzales

Printed in the U.S.A.

Dedication:

This book is dedicated to the dogs who enrich our lives—from the work they do, to the love and joy they so unselfishly give—they deserve nothing less than our love, adoration, and protection. It's equally dedicated to those who wake up each day (and stay up all night) to provide the love, shelter, training, care, and family that these wonderful critters so desperately need and deserve. To all who have opened your hearts and homes to dogs, this book is for you!

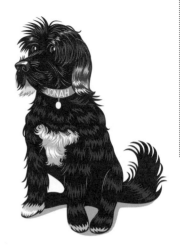

Acknowledgements:

First and foremost I'd like to thank my amazing wife and the rest of my family and friends—thank you all for your support and patience as I produced this book and continue to pursue my dreams. I promise to smile (and call) more now that the book is a reality! Thank you as well to those who have taught me—human and canine, alike—and to those who have trusted me with the care and safety of their pets. You've helped me realize my true professional passion and you drive me to continue following and perfecting it. I'd also like to extend a huge collective thank you to my book production team and to those whose generous contributions and support during my Indiegogo campaign helped to bring this book from concept to beautiful reality. Know that each and every one of you have helped me realize a dream, and that you have played an integral role in protecting the human-animal bond and the health and safety of dogs everywhere. Thank you!

Congratulations!

Whether the pup you've just added to your family is your first or your fiftieth, you've begun a fantastic journey that should bring a smile to your face each and every day. Of course, some of those days will follow sleepless nights and involve "accidents" in the house, finicky eating, rolls in "smelly stuff," and you standing in the rain waiting for your pup to pee. But those are all just part of the experience, right?

What should *not* be part of the experience though, and what this book will help you avoid, are the behavioral and digestive problems, the poisonings, illnesses, traumatic accidents, and a variety of other preventable issues and emergencies that all-too-commonly affect puppies— and indeed, dogs of all ages.

This book was born out of my mission to ensure that every new dog owner is aware of the information and advice that will get them on the right path to raising their new pup to the best of their ability, and particularly help them keep their new family member safe from serious illnesses and emergencies throughout every life stage. On these pages you will find resources, stories, and 101 of the best dog health and safety "nuggets" that I have realized and learned over my many years as a veterinarian, dog owner, husband, and father. These words of wisdom are tried and tested and have helped *many* new dog owners, just like you.

I know from experience and conversations with countless dog owners that **awareness, preparedness**, and **prevention** are the keys to providing a long, happy, healthy, and safe life for your new bundle of fur and joy. This book provides an ample dose of all three. It will serve as an invaluable resource to you and your family as you raise and care for your new pup, and see them well into their senior years.

Enjoy every minute and cherish the journey you have begun, for it truly can be one of life's most joyful and rewarding.

Sincerely,

Dr. Jason Nicholas, BVetMed(Hons)

www.ThePreventiveVet.com

Note: This book uses QR code technology to expand and enhance your learning experience. If you don't yet have a QR code reader on your smartphone, you can easily download one from your phone's app store.

Contents:

Prevent Digestive Problems

1 Go easy on the table scraps, or better still—avoid them entirely

Table scraps can easily land your pup in the hospital with a serious, and potentially fatal digestive problem. Feeding table scraps also encourages begging—which may be cute when she's a pup, but will grow old well before she does!

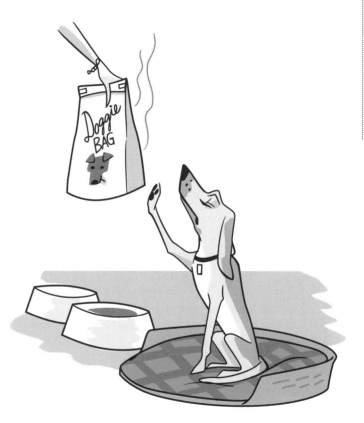

Conan, an overweight five-year-old Shih Tzu, had to spend five days in the ICU recovering from a severe and painful case of pancreatitis after he got some prime rib leftovers as a special treat. Though his hospitalization and treatment cost his owners over $3,000, they felt guilty about his condition and were ecstatic to have their beloved Conan feeling better. From the day of his discharge they worked with their veterinarian to get Conan back to a more ideal body condition and vowed to express their love for him with additional walks and cuddles.

2 Be aware of the dangers of batteries

Batteries are everywhere these days—from remote controls and children's toys to watches and even hearing aids! If your dog swallows one (or several) they can cause severe burns anywhere along her digestive tract. These types of burns often lead to an expensive surgery and prolonged hospital stay, and they can be fatal. If your pup has a habit of chewing or scavenging, be particularly careful about where you leave your battery-powered devices.

3 Be aware of the dangers of magnets

Many dogs (and children) have developed severe stomach or intestinal damage after swallowing magnets, particularly when more than one is swallowed. This type of damage is painful and debilitating, as it can lead to leakage of food and bacteria from the digestive tract. Treatment requires endoscopy or surgery, and may mean a prolonged hospital stay. If the issue isn't recognized and treated quickly, magnet ingestion can be fatal. Be aware and keep your collection of fridge magnets high up and well out of your dog's reach at all times.

4 Feed bones with great care—or ideally, not at all

All bones have the potential to break your dog's teeth and/or obstruct, irritate, or puncture her digestive tract. Any of these issues will be painful and costly, and many will land your pup on the dental or surgery table. There are safer options to satisfy your pup's innate desire for chewing. Talk to your veterinarian or a reputable trainer for recommendations.

Maximus, a four-year-old English Mastiff, occasionally got marrow bones as a treat. One day he broke a tooth while chewing on one. The fractured tooth was discovered only when he was brought to his vet two days later because he was sleeping more and not eating. Because the broken tooth was painful, and was also at increased risk of becoming infected, his owners were given the choice of having it removed by their vet or taking Maximus to a veterinary dentist for a root canal. They elected to have the broken tooth removed and forever swore off giving Maximus bones as treats.

5 Be careful where you leave presents... no matter how well they're wrapped

Wrapping paper, tape, and ribbon are no match for a dog hot on the scent of a box of chocolates or some other tasty food treat, no matter how well wrapped they are. Be careful what you leave under the tree, on countertops, or on low-lying tables. And be sure houseguests—as well as Santa Claus and the Easter Bunny—exercise the same caution.

6 Feed a complete, nutritionally-balanced, and consistent diet

Find a well-balanced diet that your pup thrives on and then stick with it. While variety may be the spice of *your* life, it can lead to frequent and uncomfortable digestive upset for your pup. This digestive distress is likely to result in multiple trips to the vet and a lot of accidents on your carpets. And an upset stomach can be very uncomfortable for your dog, so consistency in diet is best.

7 Make any food changes slowly, ideally over 1-2 weeks

If you do change your pup's diet, be sure to do so gradually. By slowly decreasing the percentage of her old food while simultaneously increasing the amount of the new, you will minimize digestive upset and spare her from uncomfortable and distressing bouts of vomiting and diarrhea.

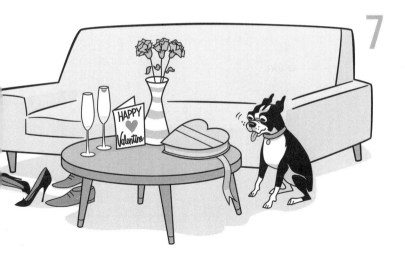

8 Keep your pup away from the kitty litter

"Kitty Roca" will not be kind to her digestive tract, and the results won't be kind to your carpets, either. Keep litter boxes behind furniture, in closets behind propped-open doors, or on elevated shelves to prevent your pup's access.

9 Keep your pup's bulk bag of dry food safely out of his reach

When given the opportunity, many dogs will eagerly gorge themselves on their kibble—they don't really have an "off," or a "hey, I'm full," switch. By properly storing your pup's bag of kibble, you'll prevent a painful and serious emergency called *food bloat* (as well as the severe case of diarrhea that typically follows it). Think about this, too, when traveling for long periods with your pup; preventing his access to the bag of food you're likely to be traveling with is yet another important reason for you to safely restrain him during travel.

Marley, a one-year-old Labrador Retriever, decided one night that his hunger couldn't wait for breakfast. He helped himself to the bag of dry food his owners stored next to his food bowl, eating about half its contents while his owners slept. He was rushed to the emergency hospital when his owners awoke to find him groaning in pain and laying on his side. He felt immediately better after anesthesia for stomach pumping and other hospital care, but his midnight buffet cost his parents $1,200 (not including a replacement bag of dog food). They are now careful to keep his food in an airtight and Marley-proof container, which they keep behind the closed door of the kitchen pantry.

10 Keep your pup away from compost

Though composting can be a great thing to do for your garden and the environment in general, it's not a great thing for your pup's digestive tract. If the food scraps in compost don't bring on a bout of vomiting and diarrhea, the bacteria and fungal toxins in there almost certainly will. Have a sturdy fence around any compost pile, keep your pup out of your garden, and don't forget about the compost pail that may be present on your kitchen counter or in the cabinet beneath your sink.

11 Watch closely when giving rawhides or compressed vegetable treats

If your dog is a "chewer," these treats will probably be fine for him. However, if he is a "gulper" or "inhaler" these treats will be neither safe nor effective. Large chunks of these treats can cause distressing and potentially fatal obstruction of your pup's digestive or respiratory systems. Additionally, if your pooch isn't thoroughly chewing these treats, he isn't getting the advertised dental benefit anyway. Monitor closely to find out which group your pup falls into and then use (or don't) accordingly.

12 Be aware of and prevent "bloat"

More properly referred to as Gastric Dilatation and Volvulus (GDV), "bloat" is a painful, serious and rapidly fatal emergency condition. Treatment typically has a high success rate, but quick recognition on your part and immediate veterinary evaluation are of the utmost importance. Certain breeds are at increased risk—including Great Danes, Doberman Pinschers, Setters, and other deep-chested breeds—especially if they come from a breeding line with a history of this condition. Several other factors can increase your dog's risk, too. Talk to your veterinarian about your pup's risk for developing GDV; and if the risk is deemed high, have your veterinarian or a board-certified surgeon do the preventive surgery at the time of your pup's spay or neuter. Please read the *Canine Bloat* blog post on our website for more information on this deadly condition, including what to watch for and how to prevent it.

Scan this QR code to learn more about GDV/Bloat.

13 Keep your pup away from your dirty laundry

Many a dollar has been spent removing socks, towels, underwear, and other garments from the stomachs and intestinal tracts of dogs. Help keep your pup off the surgery table by putting all laundry in closed hampers and keeping your pup out of the laundry room. Don't forget about the kid's room, too and be extra cautious with baby and toddler clothes, which are often stained with all manner of enticing food splatters.

14 Be aware of the dangers that pacifiers and bottle nipples can pose

These ubiquitous baby items are frequently removed from the obstructed digestive tracts of dogs all across the country. The surgical or endoscopic procedure necessary to remove them requires anesthesia and will typically set you back over $1,000. Try to pick up dropped bottle nipples promptly and consider using pacifier leashes to prevent pacifiers from hitting the ground in the first place; both can be highly effective preventive measures, and either is far cheaper for you and less distressing for your pup than the alternative!

15 In households with babies and toddlers, be sure to dispose of dirty diapers and wipes promptly and securely

These items are perhaps second only to "Kitty Roca" on the delicacy scale for many dogs. Unlike kitty roca however, expensive surgery is often necessary to remove diapers and wipes from your pooch's digestive tract. Consider putting secure diaper disposal systems or sturdy and covered wastebaskets everywhere that you might envision changing a diaper. After all, even 10 Diaper Genies® will prove less expensive than just one surgery.

Scan this QR code for more information, tips, and resources for keeping kids and pets safe around each other.

Prevent Traumas

16 Get in the habit of checking around and under your car before pulling out of your driveway or garage

Sadly, every year many dogs are inadvertently run over by those who love them the most—their owners. This is particularly common with older dogs who may not hear as well or be able to move as spritely as they once did, especially when they're basking in the sun. Make a habit of giving a quick look and pulling out slowly.

Baxter, an 11-year-old Golden Retriever, got slower in his later years and also liked to take longer and deeper naps. It was during one of these naps, on a warm summer day, that his owner backed over him as he pulled out of the garage and down the driveway. The damage to Baxter's chest was severe and, despite his owner's guilt and willingness to spend whatever it took, Baxter sadly succumbed to his injuries shortly after arriving at the ER.

17 Keep your pup inside when you're working in the yard

A hidden rock or stick can quickly become a dangerous projectile when struck by a lawnmower blade or edging string. If your pup's eye or head is in the path of that rock or stick, he's likely to suffer a painful injury. Spare him this pain and discomfort by keeping him safely inside while you, or anyone else, are laboring away in the yard.

18 Safeguard your backyard pool

Every year, many dogs die from drowning or near-drowning accidents—including some who were strong swimmers. Keep a close eye on your pup when she is swimming and know when to take her out. Install a fence around your pool to prevent her unobserved access. Pool covers, no matter how sturdy, just don't cut it—and in some cases can even make matters worse. Water surface alarms and water safety ramps are important additional tools for backyard pool safety, too.

19 Be engaged and observant at the dog park

Not every dog who goes to a dog park is well-behaved. Pay attention to how other dogs are interacting with your dog, and vice versa. If there are any concerning signs—leave. You'll avoid injuries, uncomfortable confrontations with other owners, and a host of other problems.

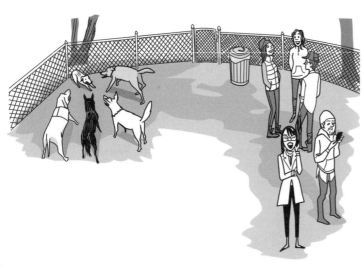

20 Sticks are not safe for a game of "fetch"

In their eager play, many dogs have run onto sticks only to be impaled in their chest, mouth, and even eyes. Many dogs have also had to undergo anesthesia and tooth extractions for stick fragments that have become lodged between their teeth or embedded under their gums. Though sticks are plentiful and (initially) free, there are far safer and better fetch toys out there. One I recommend is the Kong® Safestix—safe, easy to clean, and dogs love it.

21 Don't let your dog and small child swim together without very close supervision

Either can quickly drown or nearly drown the other. If you can't be present with them when they're swimming together, don't let them do so at all. It truly isn't worth the risk.

22 Use a doggie life jacket (PFD) when your pup swims in a river, lake, or ocean

Even if she is a strong swimmer, your pup can easily become exhausted and drown in rough conditions or a strong current. PFDs are also a safety must if your pooch spends time on a boat or if she rides the waves on a surfboard or stand-up paddleboard. Companies like Ruff Wear® and EzyDog® make some great (and stylish) life jackets for dogs.

23 Learn to recognize rip currents at the ocean, and never let your dog swim near one

Warning signs for these deadly currents will often, though not always, be posted on beaches with lifeguards. However, not all beaches are guarded and not all rip currents are marked. Learn to recognize and avoid them—both for your dog and for yourself. Not only have dogs drowned in riptides, but so too have distressed owners who have jumped in to try and save them. See the rip current article on the website for the National Oceanic & Atmospheric Association (ripcurrents. noaa.gov).

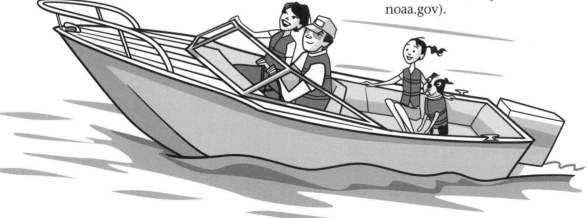

24 Improve your pup's nighttime visibility

It's tough for drivers to avoid hitting what they can't see. Using reflective or self-illuminating collars, leashes, and clothing on walks with your pup between dusk and dawn will help ensure that your puppy *and you* are seen and safe. There are lots of great light-up products for dogs on the market; you can read reviews of several of them on our website.

Maddie, a six-year-old Wheaton Terrier, was out on her evening walk with her dad when she bolted into the street after a cat. The driver who hit her had no way of seeing her, and said he hadn't even known that there was a dog in the road until he realized he had hit something. Fortunately for Maddie and her family, the driver wasn't going very fast and she was struck on her back end—avoiding the head and chest trauma that often accompanies such accidents. She suffered a few broken bones in one of her back legs and was peeing blood for the next several days. But after her surgery, hospital stay, and the ensuing eight-week period of crate rest (to allow her surgically-repaired leg to fully heal), she was back to her energetic old self—with one exception. Maddie now wears a blinking collar, reflective jacket, and a leash on all of her nightly walks.

25 Be aware of the dangers of electrical cords and power cables

The shock your pup can get from chewing on these cords will not only cause burns in his mouth, but it can also lead to seizures and fluid build-up in his lungs. Electric cord shock is painful, debilitating, expensive, and potentially fatal. It can be prevented with awareness, cord covers, and safe positioning of your pup's crate. Electric cord shock is most common in young puppies and in dogs of any age with separation anxiety.

26 Be aware around rocking chairs and recliners

An ill-placed paw, tail, or head can easily be crushed by the weight of a rocking chair or closing recliner. Always be mindful of where your pup is before you sit down, rock, or stretch out. An important tip for nursing moms: though it might be difficult to do in your state of perpetual exhaustion, this is one to keep in mind when using a glider or rocking chair late at night or in the wee hours of the morning.

27 Be aware of the dangers of escalators

If you take your dog on an escalator or moving sidewalk she should *always* be in your arms for the *entire* trip. If she's too big to be in your arms, or if your hands are too full, then, for her safety, find another way to get between floors. And there are always safer alternatives—stairs, elevators, or leaving her at home. Escalators and moving sidewalks can and have caused painful, distressing, and disfiguring injuries to dogs who have been unfortunate enough to get their paws, ears, or leashes caught in the end plate teeth. Carry or avoid—always.

28 Be aware of the dangers of home office paper shredders

Curious or ill-placed tongues, tails, and ears can shred just as easily in some machines as paper. Be safe—keep paper shredders unplugged and off the floor. Whatever you do, never leave your office paper shredder in the *stand-by* or *automatic* position.

29 In late summer and early fall be aware of the dangers of foxtails and other grass seeds

If your pup is sneezing excessively, shaking her head, squinting with either or both eyes, or limping after a run through a tall grass field, bring her to your veterinarian to see if an embedded foxtail might be responsible. Left undetected or untreated, grass seeds can cause significant, painful, and expensive problems. Avoid unkempt tall grass fields in the summer to protect your pup. If these fields are unavoidable, look into and use the field guard by OutFox® (OutFoxFieldGuard.com) and a good pair of dog booties.

30 Keep your pup well back from the curb when waiting to cross at an intersection

Have you ever noticed all the tire marks on curbs at intersections? It takes only one person to cut their turn too tight to result in your pup's injury or death. The milliseconds you may save in being that much closer to the curb, and crossing the street sooner just aren't worth it. Wait with your dog just a couple steps back to prevent a heart-breaking accident.

31 Avoid choke chains, pinch collars, and dangling ID tags on dogs who spend time on decks or in crates

Dogs have died from strangulation in their panic and struggle to free themselves when the loop on their choke chain or pinch collar, or their dangling ID tags, have gotten caught between deck slats or between the wires of their crate. Choke chains and pinch collars should be used only as control aids when out walking—if at all. They should *never* be used as everyday, around-the-clock neckwear. Consider ID tags that lie flat against your pup's collar to keep him safe while still keeping him identifiable.

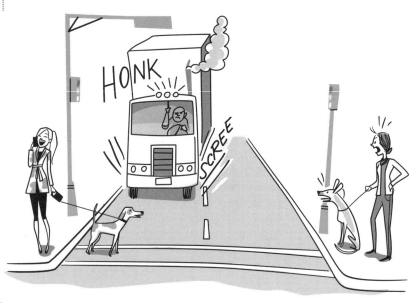

32 Prevent fighting amongst your own dogs

This is especially important when introducing a new dog (puppy or adult) into your household. This can happen when everyone's getting to know each other, or when food, treats, or a favorite toy are involved. Dog crates, sturdy baby gates, and basket muzzles can save your dogs a lot of pain and suffering, while saving you heartbreak, stress, time, and money. If fighting proves to be a persistent problem, speak with a veterinary behaviorist or a reputable and certified dog trainer. Information about behaviorists and trainers can be found on the *Resources* page of our website.

33 Don't let your pup ride with her head out the window

Not only can kicked-up rocks and other flying road debris injure her eyes, ears, nose, throat, or skull, but one short stop or a passing squirrel can send her flying out of the car. It's okay to open the windows a bit, but not enough for her to get her head out—*even* if she's wearing eye protection.

34 Following any surgery, be sure to appropriately restrict your pup's exercise for the period of time recommended by your vet

Too quick a return to exercise and play following many surgeries can result in surgical failure, infections, and bleeding that can land your pup back on the surgery table, prolong her recovery, and cost you additional time, money, and stress. Talk to your veterinarian about exercise restriction recommendations, and sedation, if necessary. This is another reason to introduce your pup to crate training early on in life.

35 Routinely check around your growing puppy's neck, tail, limbs, and muzzle

Puppies grow into dogs quickly, and your vigilance will ensure that no rubber bands, string, ribbons, or outgrown collars become embedded in their skin. Removal of such embedded material would require sedation or anesthesia for necessary surgery. This tip is particularly important if you have young kids living in or visiting your home, as they often love to decorate puppies with these cute but dangerous fashion accessories.

36 Don't use scissors to cut mats, gum, paint, or anything else out of your pup's coat

It's often hard to know where the mat or stuck material ends and your pup's skin begins—and one wrong guess can result in a bloody and painful cut. Opt for an electric beard trimmer instead and work slowly. Alternatively, bring your dog to your vet or a professional groomer to have the offending material removed. Any of these options will be less likely to result in a painful (and potentially expensive) cut.

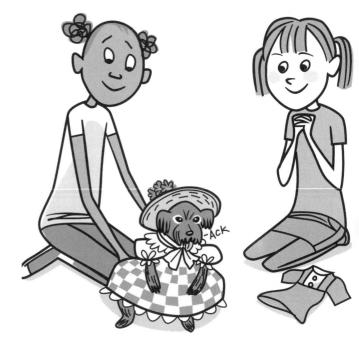

Prevent Toxicities

37 Hang purses, diaper bags, backpacks, and all other bags far out of your pup's reach

Our bags often contain a variety of substances and products that are toxic or otherwise hazardous to our dogs. Don't risk your pup's health and safety—or that of your bank account, either. Hanging your bag or purse from the back of a chair or from a doorknob typically isn't safe enough, and neither is dropping it on a sofa, table, or countertop. Getting in the habit of hanging all bags from wall hooks, coat racks, or behind closet doors is the best way to keep your pup truly safe. And don't forget to ensure that all babysitters, houseguests, and other visitors take the same simple precaution.

Bowser, a four-year-old Boxer, decided to help himself to the dirty diaper that was left in the diaper bag after his family's long day out at the park. The bag was left hanging from the back of the stroller—easy pickings for Bowser. Two days later, Bowser's energy level dropped, and he started vomiting. He was brought to the hospital, where a gelatinous mass of diaper material blocking the passage of food from Bowser's stomach to his intestines was found at surgery. His little forage into the diaper bag not only created a big mess on the living room carpet, but it also cost the family more than $3,000 in veterinary bills. Bowser recovered well and fully, and now his owners are careful to hang the diaper bag (and all others) on the wall hooks they promptly installed in their entry hallway.

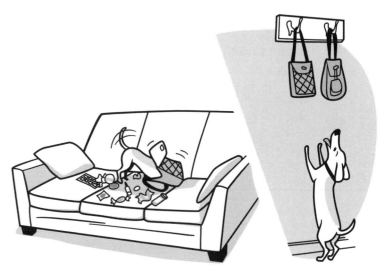

38 Truly be aware of the dangers of chocolate

Though many pet owners are seemingly aware of the dangers of chocolate in dogs, chocolate toxicity remains one of the most common poisonings seen at veterinary hospitals and called into pet poison control hotlines. Keep your dogs out of the kitchen when baking with chocolate and recognize that no amount of wrapping paper and tape will prevent your pup from sniffing out and eating a gifted box of these yummy treats. Be particularly careful around the holidays, and ask any gift-bearing guests to do the same. The higher the cocoa content, the worse and more potent the chocolate toxicity effects are. If your dog does eat chocolate (including garden cocoa mulch), call your vet, local animal ER, or a pet poison control hotline immediately. If she is already anxious, panting, or having seizures skip the phone call and bring her immediately for veterinary attention.

39 Never self-prescribe medications or supplements for your pup

Medications and supplements should be given to your pup *only* on the advice of a veterinarian. Even if you are a human pharmacist, medical doctor, or nurse, you must heed this advice if you want to avoid an inadvertent poisoning. Safety for people, even for babies, does not equal safety for dogs and many people have unintentionally poisoned, sickened, and even killed their own dogs by self-prescribing. This point cannot be stressed enough—don't self-prescribe. Check with a veterinarian first.

40 Don't store medications or supplements on countertops, tables, or nightstands

"Counter surfing" should be an Olympic sport for many dogs. Even if your pup doesn't have this habit, there are still lots of ways for these pills and bottles to wind up on the floor. Think about the family cat walking on the counter—perhaps she really is trying to poison your new pup. Also think about your early morning swat at the alarm clock in search of the snooze button—if you store medicine or supplement bottles on that nightstand they're likely to go flying. Protect your pup by storing all medications and supplements safely behind closed cabinet doors. That way, none of your pets will have access and pills are less likely to wind up on the floor.

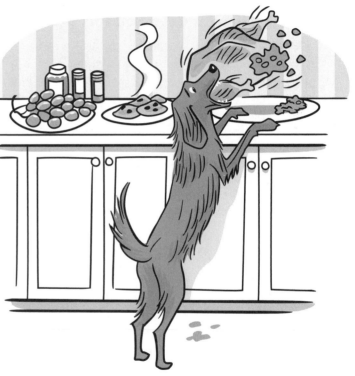

41 Get in the habit of dispensing <u>all</u> medications and supplements over a sink or bowl

Your pup won't have a chance to gobble up a pill that drops into a confined space (like the sink or a big bowl), but there's a good chance she'll beat you to the one that hits the floor. It's equally likely that she'll find the one that rolls under the couch before you do. Regardless of whether it's her medication/supplement or yours, dispensing it over a sink or bowl is easy to do and will help you keep her safe from one of the most common pet emergencies—poisoning.

Hamish, a six-year-old Scotty, didn't hesitate when several of his owner's prescription pills fell out of her hand and on to the floor while she was taking them one night before bed. Fortunately for Hamish, his owner didn't hesitate either and quickly called animal poison control. She got the information necessary to handle the problem at home and learned what to monitor for that would warrant a trip to the ER.

Hamish was fortunately unaffected, but his owner now keeps all of her medications stored safely in the bathroom cabinet and always dispenses them over the sink.

42 Be aware of the dangers of uncooked yeast bread dough

Your pup's stomach is an ideal proofing oven. If he were to eat uncooked yeast bread dough the yeast would activate, causing the dough to rise in his stomach. The result would be a painful build up of gas and alcohol that could lead to stomach bloat, digestive obstruction, alcohol poisoning, and even death. Don't give him the opportunity. Leave all bread dough to rise on an elevated shelf, in the microwave, or in the oven—not on the kitchen counter or table. This is an uncommon and little-known emergency, but it's very important to be aware of it, especially around the holidays, because it can be very severe when it happens.

43 Be aware of the dangers of macadamia nuts

Not only can macadamia nuts cause obstruction of your pup's digestive tract, they can cause a toxicity that will temporarily prevent her from using her back legs. If the macadamias are covered in chocolate, as they so often are, the problems will be even worse—see also *Dangers of chocolate* tip.

44 Stay away from xylitol

Xylitol is a sweetener that's gaining in popularity because of its anti-cavity properties for people and its benefits for human diabetics. However xylitol is *deadly* for dogs. Even a small amount can drop your pup's blood sugar and destroy her liver. Look for xylitol in gums, mints, chewable vitamins, toothpastes, mouthwashes, baked goods, sugar substitutes, and a variety of other products. Take the necessary (and often simple) steps—such as safely hanging your purse and other bags—to keep all sources of xylitol well out of your pup's reach.

45 Appreciate that "childproof" does not equal "petproof"

Dogs aren't so subtle as to try to twist the cap off a bottle of medication. No cap or pill vial, childproof or not, will keep your pup 100% safe. Your best line of defense is a safe location for all pill bottles. Bear this in mind when putting down a bottle of pills—is it *truly* out of your pup's reach? If it isn't you're putting her at unnecessary risk of poisoning.

46 Keep your pups away from your garden after planting or digging up bulbs

The bulbs of daffodils, tulips, narcissus, irises, and many other common spring flowers can cause problems ranging from skin irritation and gastro-intestinal upset to organ failure and death in dogs who eat them. Don't allow your dogs to dig them up once planted and be sure to keep these bulbs well out of your pup's reach when stored.

47 Be aware of the dangers of antifreeze

If it contains ethylene glycol—which most anti-freeze does—even a few licks can give your dog a debilitating, expensive, and potentially fatal case of acute kidney failure. Properly store all anti-freeze containers, promptly clean up all spills and leaks, and consider using a *safer* propylene glycol-based alternative instead. Many hardware and auto care stores carry these alternative, pet-safer* formulas—just ask!

No antifreeze is pet-safe, but the propylene glycol-based ones are certainly safer than those with ethylene glycol.

48 Be aware of the potential dangers of grapes, raisins, and currants

Consumption of even a small amount of one of these fruits may be enough to cause a debilitating (and potentially fatal) case of acute kidney fail-ure for your pup. Recognize that grapes, raisins, and currants are found in a variety of common products—including trail mix, bread/bagels, and cookies—and that they are, on their own, com-mon toddler snacks, which often wind up on the ground.

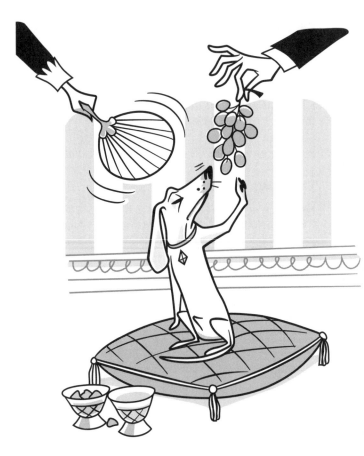

49 Be aware of the dangers of rat and mouse poisons—both at home and on the road

These compounds are designed to kill, and they don't discriminate between your dog and the rodents you are targeting. There are many types available, and the toxicity of some can be significantly stronger, and more difficult to treat, than others. Research carefully, follow all label instructions, and be extremely careful where you deploy and store these poisons. Consider using a reputable exterminator to explore pet-safe methods of rodent control rather than doing it yourself, or try nature's rodenticide: a cat! Be aware of the dangers of rodenticides also when walking your pup around a city park, traveling with your pup, and when moving into a new apartment or home. When traveling or moving with your pup, always ask if rodenticides are in use, and make removal of them a condition of any rental or home purchase agreement.

50 Be aware that many plants and flowers can be dangerous to dogs

There's a good chance that some of the plants and flowers in and around your home right now could seriously sicken or even kill your puppy. Knowing what's safe and what's potentially dangerous is an important step in safeguarding your new pup's health and safety. You can find the ASPCA toxic and non-toxic plant list on our website. This fantastic resource is easy to use and is compiled, maintained, and updated by the toxicology experts at the ASPCA Animal Poison Control Center. For those with smartphones, both the ASPCA and Pet Poison Helpline have excellent pet poison apps available for download.

51 Be aware of the dangers of sago palms and other cycads

Whether they are part of your outdoor landscaping or kept as houseplants, even a small nibble on these plants is likely to be deadly for your dog. The toxins in them are extremely harmful to your pup's liver. Be aware of this when traveling with your dogs, too—especially to warmer climates where these plants are more likely to be found thriving outdoors.

52 Be aware of the danger of certain mushrooms

Not all mushrooms are edible, and certain ones can be deadly. Of particular concern are those in the *Amanita* genus. Use caution on hikes and check your yard regularly to prevent your pup's exposure. There are lots of good resources for mushroom identification both in your local bookstore and online—we list and link to some of them on the *Resources* page of our website.

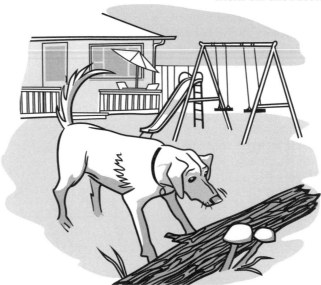

53 Be aware of the dangers of rock salt and other ice melts

If your pup licks enough of an ice melt from his paws following a winter walk, you're both likely to be in for a long night. Many ice melts can lead to digestive upset resulting in vomiting and diarrhea. If you know that your sidewalks or roads are treated, be sure to thoroughly rinse off your dog's paws after your walk or consider protecting their paws with dog-specific booties.

54 Be aware of the dangers of and learn to recognize blue-green algae

Common in lakes and ponds, the toxins in these types of algae can lead to problems ranging from skin irritation to liver failure, and can be fatal. Blooms are most common from summer to fall, but can also occur at other times of the year. Each state's veterinary service or Department of Health will typically post on their website when blooms are seen or expected, as well as photos and descriptions so you can learn to recognize and avoid them.

55 Be aware of the dangers of snail and slug bait

Most snail and slug baits contain a compound called metaldehyde, a chemical that is *highly* toxic to dogs. Unfortunately, these baits are often formulated with molasses too, making them even more enticing to your inquisitive pup. Ideally, try to use non-chemical types of snail and slug control instead—such as copper strips, crushed egg shells, or beer poured into a tuna can. If you must use chemicals though, consider the pet-safer option of an iron phosphate-based product. Just be aware that even the iron phosphate-based products pose a toxic risk to your pets if they ingest enough of it.

56 Be aware of the dangers of rattlesnakes

If you live in or routinely hike with your pooch in an area where rattlesnakes are common, look into avoidance training and discuss the use of the rattlesnake vaccine with your veterinarian. A rattlesnake bite is a serious and debilitating emergency. The venom's toxin is painful and can prove rapidly fatal. If your pup is bitten, vaccinated or not, an immediate trip to the veterinarian is of the utmost importance. Please read the blog posts on rattlesnake avoidance training methods and rattlesnake bites on The Preventive Vet website.

57 Be aware of the dangers of Bufo toads

A single lick from your pup to one of these toads can be deadly. Find out if Bufo toads are present in your town or in areas where you plan to travel or hike with your pup. If so, take extra precautions to keep him well away from these dangerous toads and know what to do in the event he does get a lick in.

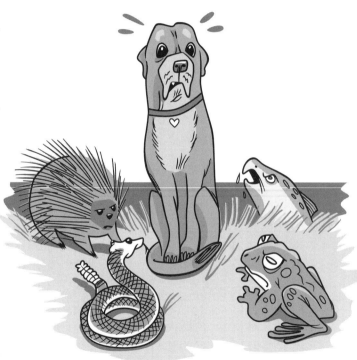

Prevent Disease or Recognize it Earlier

58 Research your puppy's breed(s) and be aware of their medical predispositions

Some medical conditions and illnesses are more likely to occur in certain breeds, these are known as *breed predispositions*. In some cases, prior knowledge of them can help you reduce their effects or even prevent them entirely. This little bit of research can protect your puppy from discomfort and illness, and save you time and money in the long run. Speak with your veterinarian and breeder.

59 Protect your pup with appropriate vaccines

While *every* dog doesn't need *every* vaccine, they *all* need *certain ones*. Vaccines are about the health and well-being of your dog, as well as that of all the other dogs in your community. And in the case of some vaccines—such as leptospirosis and rabies—immunizing your dog protects you and the other people in your home and community as well. Speak with your veterinarian to determine which vaccines your dog should have, and at what intervals.

60 Use safe and effective parasite prevention <u>year-round</u>

Heartworm disease sickens and kills many dogs every year—fortunately, it is easily preventable. Fleas, ticks, and some of the common intestinal parasites which affect dogs can cause disease in people, too. But these are also often preventable. Consistent use of effective preventatives will keep your pup free from fleas, ticks, heartworms and intestinal worms—safeguarding the health of *everyone* in your family. Talk to your veterinarian about recommended products and visit the website for the Companion Animal Parasite Council (CAPCVet.org) for more information. To learn about fleas and all the reasons why you should keep them at bay, please read the flea blog post on our website.

61 Don't skip wellness veterinary visits

Visits to the vet aren't *just* about vaccines—in fact, in many cases, they're not about vaccines at all. The importance of a good physical examination and discussion with your vet cannot be overstated. Remember, just because your dog *looks* healthy to you doesn't necessarily mean that he is healthy. Prevention and early detection are crucial steps to a long and healthy life for your pup.

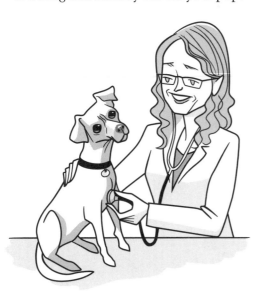

62 Bathe your dog regularly as needed and brush her coat frequently

Some basic grooming will not only keep your pup's coat clean and free of mats and certain parasites, but it will help you with early detection of wounds, swellings, and potentially cancerous growths, too. Brushing and combing also helps decrease stress—both for you and your dog.

63 Get your pup accustomed to you touching and evaluating her teeth, ears, and paws

Not only will this make her at-home routine care easier, it will also greatly reduce the stress she'll experience in your veterinarian's office and at the groomer. As an added bonus, it will help you detect problems earlier and may make the treatment of those problems easier and less expensive.

64 Check your pup's ears regularly

Ear infections are consistently among the top reasons people bring their dogs to the veterinarian. Sadly, they often do so only after the infection is well established and has already caused their dog significant discomfort. A quick weekly look and sniff will spare your pup discomfort and save you money. Have your veterinarian, or one of their technicians, teach you what to look for and show you how to safely and effectively clean your pup's ears.

65 Brush your pup's teeth frequently

Imagine the state of *your* mouth if you never brushed your teeth. Brushing your dog's teeth is often easy and can make a big difference in his dental and general health! The earlier you get your pup used to this, the easier it'll be. Talk to your veterinarian about a demonstration and about safe and effective at-home options for your dog's dental care.

66 Keep an eye on your pup's energy level, eliminations, thirst, and appetite

Changes in any of these, even if subtle, can be an indication of illness. The more regularly you monitor, the more likely you are to detect these changes. And the earlier you detect and act on a problem, the easier it is likely to be on your pup (and potentially your pocketbook).

67 Be aware of Salmon Poisoning Disease

Exclusive to the Pacific Northwest of the U.S., and certain parts of British Columbia, Salmon Poisoning Disease can be a debilitating and potentially fatal condition for your pup. If you fish or bring your dog to the river in these parts of the world, this is an important condition for you to know about. Early recognition and treatment is imperative for quick and effective treatment.

68 Be aware of and prevent heat stroke

Heat stroke is a debilitating and easily avoidable emergency. It's truly horrible and often fatal. Heat stroke happens most frequently (but by no means exclusively) to dogs left in parked cars and those exercised too vigorously on hot days. It most commonly affects the brachycephalic (short-nosed) breeds, such as bulldogs, boxers, and shih tzus. However, *all* breeds and mixes are susceptible. Because of their decreased ability to regulate their body temperature, puppies and older dogs are also at increased risk. For more information—including additional risk factors and advice for avoiding this horrific condition—please read the heat stroke blog post on our website.

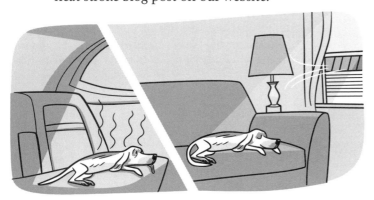

Sally, a seven-year-old Standard Poodle, was rushed into the emergency hospital after she collapsed from heat stroke in her owner's car. The windows were cracked while her owners ran into the store, but it was an unseasonably warm day in the low 80s. Despite very aggressive treatments and support, Sally's blood clotting system failed. Her prognosis was grave, and Sally's family had to make the heart-wrenching decision to euthanize her. Sally was alone in the car for just 20 minutes.

Please scan this QR code to visit the "I Hate Heat Stroke" campaign page and learn what you can do to prevent this devastating and easily avoidable condition.

Prevent Multiple Problems

69 Fence your yard

Yard fences aren't only about keeping your dogs in; they keep other dogs (and wildlife) out, too. Both functions are important to prevent some very expensive, very painful, and potentially fatal emergencies. A fence is an important investment if you plan to let your pup out in the yard without a leash. It's important to recognize that while electric fences may do a great job of keeping your dog in the yard, they provide no protection against other dogs and animals coming in.

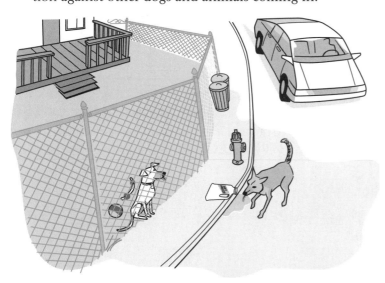

70 Provide your pup with a pet-safe area inside your home

This area can be his crate or any quiet room that's off limits to houseguests and children. Having this space is particularly important around the holidays, during parties, when you have overnight visitors, and when you bring a new baby into the house. This one precaution can prevent toxicities, cases of vomiting and diarrhea, soiling of your guest's belongings, escape from the house, bites to children, and a host of other problems. It's best to get your dog comfortable in this area as a puppy and reacquaint him to it frequently and well in advance of any likely stressful event.

71 Buckle up pup for the drive

Be it a crate, carrier, or travel harness, proper dog travel restraint will keep not only your pets safe, it will do the same for you, your family, and everyone else on the road as well. Restraint decreases your dog's risk of injury or death in the event of an accident or short stop, it decreases your chances of an accident in the first place, and it also prevents your pup from jumping through an open window or getting to the contents of your purse while you're not looking. Safely restraining your puppy is easy to do and there are several good and effective options available. The key is to choose a product that has been tested and to *use it for every trip,* no matter how short and no matter how calm your pup is in the car. You can find lots more information about pet travel restraint, including reviews of products, on our website.

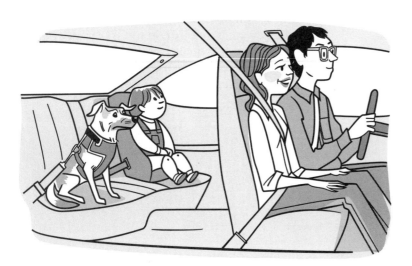

Scotch, a Labrador Retriever, was four years old when he jumped out of an open window in the family car as it sat at a stop sign only three blocks from his house. The family didn't see the squirrel he was likely chasing, but they did see the passing car that hit him as he ran through the intersection. Scotch suffered brain swelling, multiple rib fractures, and internal bleeding as a result of his accident. He did survive, but he needed a full eight days in the ICU to do so. He now wears a travel harness every time he goes for a ride, no matter how short or long the trip.

72 Don't allow your pup to roam free around the neighborhood

Even if she's lucky enough to avoid getting hit and killed by a car, and manages to avoid eating something toxic (antifreeze, rat poison, slug bait, or any of the other common outdoor poisons) your neighbors probably won't be too pleased with her defecating on their lawn or digging up their garden. For her safety, and for harmony within your neighborhood, don't let your pup roam free.

73 Don't leave your dog outside or walk her off-leash around July 4th, New Year's Eve, or any other time fireworks are expected

Fireworks and other loud noises (such as thunder) are no fun for dogs. The anxiety and fear these noises create frequently cause outdoor dogs to escape yards and run off, putting them at risk of getting lost, hit by a car, or otherwise injured. Every year July 5th proves to be the busiest day in pet shelters all across the country. Protect your pup by keeping her inside when fireworks are expected. If you *must* take her out, be sure to keep her on leash with a well-fitted collar (or harness) and ensure that her identification is visible and up-to-date. If your pup proves particularly noise phobic, speak to your veterinarian about behavioral modification techniques and/or sedation, and consider trying the Thundershirt™ (Thunder-Shirt.com) to decrease her anxiety.

74 Don't let your toddler or any other young child be the only one holding onto your pup's leash while on a walk

Cute as this situation may seem and as much as your child may protest, the sudden appearance of a squirrel, cat, or other enticing object can quickly cause your dog to bolt, landing your child face down on the ground or even worse, in front of a passing car. Always ensure that a responsible adult has one of their hands securely on the leash at all times, as well.

41

75 Understand and take the necessary precautions to prevent bolting

If your dog runs out of an opening door (bolts)—be it the front door of your house, a car door, or any other—there is a real risk that he will be hit by a car and suffer severe and potentially fatal injuries. Training, sturdy baby gates, dog crates, and ensuring that you have a good grip on his leash prior to opening the car door are just some steps you can take that will go a long way toward preventing this risky behavior.

76 Have your pup spayed/neutered

This procedure prevents more than just unintended pregnancies. It can tame undesirable behaviors, prevent certain diseases and emergencies, and make the treatment of some chronic conditions easier. Speak with your veterinarian about the procedure and about recommended timing. Even for breeding dogs, this is still an important procedure to have done once their breeding days are behind them.

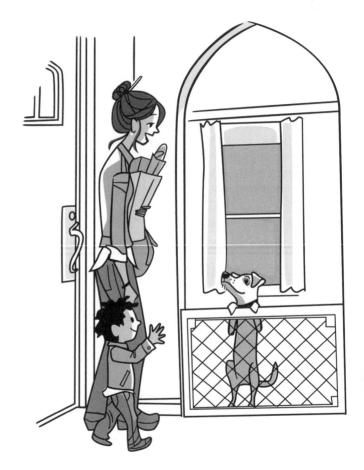

77 Work with a good trainer

This small, early investment will pay off in many aspects of your pup's happiness, health, safety, and overall wellness. And it'll make your life far easier in the long run, too. Use a trainer who focuses on positive reinforcement, desensitization, counter conditioning, and other methods that are well-grounded in behavioral science. Avoid those who profess and subscribe to dominance theory. Talk to your veterinarian and see the *Pet Behavior* and *Training* links on the *Resources* page of our website.

78 Provide plenty of interaction and play time

For most dogs, a little extra "you time" is better than any food treat. Time spent together can go a long way toward decreasing stress—both yours and his. These interactions not only improve your dog's health and weight, but they can also help prevent or correct certain behavioral problems.

79 Don't skip the puppy socialization classes

The first three months of your puppy's life are the most crucial for her social skill development. Taking advantage of this period and helping her get comfortable with a variety of people, pets, sights, and sounds can go a long way toward preventing a host of behavioral problems later in life. Read the position statement on puppy socialization from the American Veterinary Society of Animal Behavior (AVSAB) and talk to your veterinarian to ensure that your pup receives at least her first vaccinations and deworming of their puppy series in time to start a puppy socialization class before she is 12 weeks old.

Scan this QR code to visit the "Behavior and Training Resources" page on The Preventive Vet website.

80 Request that all overnight visitors keep the doors to their room and bathroom securely closed at all times

Though they don't do so intentionally, house-guests often bring any number of pet toxins and other hazards into your home in their suitcases, toiletry kits, purses, and jackets. Keeping those items off the floor and preventing your pup's access to these rooms will go a long way to keeping her safe and healthy.

Shelby, an adorable 10-month-old Labrador Retriever puppy, needed an endoscopic procedure to remove the underwear she had eaten from the luggage of the aunt who was visiting for the holidays. As many overnight visitors will do, the aunt put her dirty clothes in her empty suitcase, which sat on the floor in the guest-room. Shelby's dietary adventures cost her family over $800 and almost ruined their holiday plans. Now the door to the guestroom stays closed whenever visitors come to stay, and Shelby's family is careful to keep their own laundry in a covered hamper in the laundry room, as well.

81 Get your pup used to a head collar, muzzle, harness, and crate early on in life

These aren't just great training tools, they're great safety aids, too. Many of the most common pet toxicities, injuries, and other emergencies can easily be prevented if you use these tools correctly. Talk with your veterinarian or a good trainer for advice on correct sizing and use.

82 Be careful how and where you store your fishing gear

Many people have inadvertently "caught" their dog, even when they're not actively fishing. We in the veterinary emergency world have all seen dogs that have swallowed or been impaled by fishing hooks while trying to lick off the remnants of bait or a recent catch. These injuries typically require sedation for removal of the hook, and some even require expensive surgery. Protect your pup and your wallet; keep your tackle boxes and fishing rods well out of reach whether out on the river or in your garage.

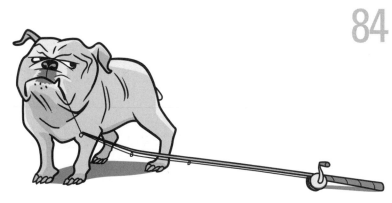

83 Prevent "counter surfing"

Don't know what this is? Picture a dog standing on his hind legs, nose sweeping across the table or counter, and you've got "counter surfing." (Alternatively, you can look at the illustration on page 23 for an example.) If you know that your dog has an inclination for this sport, keep him out of the kitchen and bathrooms. As an added precaution, make sure that dangerous items are kept off nightstands, tables and countertops—even if you think they're out of your pup's reach. After all, what good athlete doesn't like to strive for a new personal best?

84 Use child safety locks on cabinets when necessary

Though your pup may not have opposable thumbs, she may be (or may become) quite handy with her nose and paws. Installing child safety locks on low cabinets where food, trash, medicines, or chemicals are stored is an easy way to keep her safe from a variety of toxins and other potentially life-threatening hazards.

85 Appreciate <u>all</u> the benefits of using a leash

Leashes aren't *just* about preventing painful, expensive, and often fatal hit-by-car traumas. They can prevent poisonings, dogfights, lawsuits, and a host of other problems, too. Regular use of a leash is one of the best, and one of the easiest steps you can take to guard your pup's health, and safety, and give you peace of mind. Just be careful of and avoid the use of retractable leashes—these pose their own set of dangers to both pets and people.

Maggie, a three-year-old Daschund, was brought to the hospital because of difficulty breathing she was experiencing two days after a late night off-leash walk with her owner around a city park. It was determined that the breathing difficulties were a result of the blood that had built up in her lungs from the rat poison she had eaten while in that park. Thanks to vitamin K replacement, oxygen supplementation, blood transfusions and other intensive care, she's okay. However, her treatment cost her family almost $5,000 and a lot of distress. Maggie's status was touch-and-go and she had to be away from her family and littermate brother for four days. Following Maggie's brush with death, her owners became strong believers in the importance of leashes and took a more proactive approach to learning about all the poisons and other hazards that could harm their dogs.

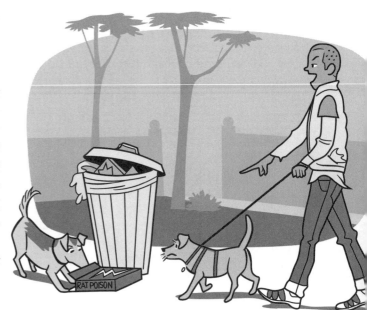

86 Keep your pup's nails well trimmed

Not only do torn nails bleed (a lot), but long nails can make walking painful and can *grow* into your dog's feet and pads. Ouch! Ask your veterinarian's staff or your groomer to show you how to safely trim your dog's nails, or just let them do it regularly. An important point is to take this process slowly—be careful and be patient! If you cut too short (known as "quicking") once, he isn't likely to forget it any time soon.

87 Be careful with your dog's weight

Obesity in dogs has become an epidemic. It puts them at increased risk for a variety of chronic illnesses—such as arthritis, skin infections, high blood pressure, and heart disease, and it increases their risk for certain emergencies: cruciate tears, heat stroke, severe pancreatitis, etc. Dogs don't have opposable thumbs, so if you store their food correctly and practice restraint with the treats you can help your pup achieve and maintain a healthy body condition. Monitor your dog's weight and body condition regularly and talk to your veterinarian to determine the number of calories your dog should be receiving each day.

Miles, a lovable nine-year-old Westie, was attacked by the neighbor's dog one sunny summer afternoon. He suffered several bite wounds that required surgical repair. He did well for the first three days following surgery, but because he had "let his figure go" a bit over the years, he had lots of fat under his skin. Though this excessive fat likely prevented the bites from reaching his abdominal cavity, it also complicated his recovery. A second, more aggressive surgery was eventually needed to remove the dead fat tissue that was preventing his wounds from healing. Miles eventually recovered from his ordeal, and his owners accepted the fact that they had been overfeeding him. They got him started on a weight loss program designed by their vet. And though Miles still carries a few extra pounds, he's nowhere near the "ottoman" he once was. Shortly after this ordeal, his owners had a fence installed around their yard.

88 Use sturdy, covered trash cans and wastebaskets <u>throughout</u> your home— and consider further securing them behind closed cabinet or closet doors

Your trash is your dog's feast, but it may prove a sickening one. Food scraps and wrappers, as well as used feminine hygiene products and dirty diapers, are particularly enticing to most dogs, and especially hazardous. Taking the simple step of covering and securing your trash cans and wastebaskets can save you both a lot of pain and trouble—as well as a trip to the animal ER.

Zelda, a 12-year-old Jack Russell Terrier, had a habit of sneaking things from the trash for extra snacks. When she was younger, her owners quickly learned the importance of securing the trash cans and wastebaskets in the house and of being diligent not to put anything too enticing in the smaller wastebaskets. Sadly, while Zelda's owners were traveling, the pet sitter forgot these important steps and discarded something of interest in the bathroom wastebasket. It's difficult to say exactly when Zelda got to it, but after three days of vomiting and lethargy she was brought into the clinic suffering from shock. Zelda had an obstructed and leaky bowel, and despite aggressive stabilization and referral to a local pet ER/ICU, she never made it on to the surgery table. Her condition was too critical and Zelda suffered cardiac arrest and passed away while being prepped for emergency surgery.

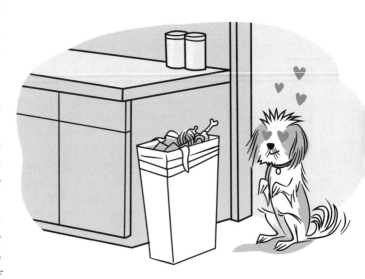

Be Prepared for Emergencies

89 Have your pup microchipped

This simple procedure can prove an important step to help reunite you with your dog should it become lost or stolen. Though the ideal time to have your pup chipped is when it is getting spayed or neutered, any other time is just fine. Be sure to register the chip, keep your contact information up to date, and have your veterinarian scan the chip for proper function and placement each time you bring your dog into their office.

90 Identification tags are important, and they're changing with the times

Because they're so easy to see and read, tags are one of the most effective ways to identify lost dogs. Be sure to include your pup's name and your cell phone number, at the very least. If you can fit them, an email address and an indication of whether your dog has a chronic medical condition are also good details to include. Better still: check out the QR code ID tags made by PetHub (www.PetHub.com) for a newer and better twist on the traditional dog tag.

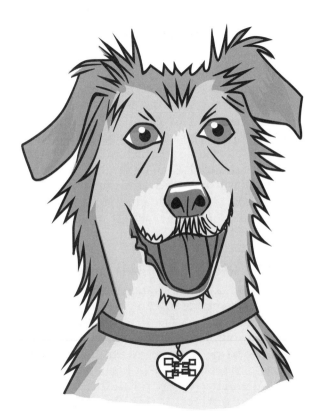

91 Include your pup in your family's emergency preparedness plans

If a natural disaster strikes and evacuation is necessary, you don't want to leave your pup behind and you can't afford to spend precious time scrambling to figure out who's leashing up the dogs, where the leashes are, etc. Create an evacuation plan that includes your pets, and make sure you have a place to go which will accept your dog. A little advanced planning can help prevent panic, which in turn decreases stress and improves *everybody's* chances for survival. See the *Disaster Preparedness for Pets* checklist available for free download on our website.

92 Take a pet first aid class

Not every accident or emergency is preventable and, in many cases, knowing what to do (and what *not* to do) for first aid can have a big impact on your pup's comfort and survival. Check with your local pet emergency hospital or humane society to see if they offer first aid classes, many do. Alternatively, check with the American Red Cross or private pet first aid companies. Just remember, first aid is often just that… *first* aid. In many cases a veterinarian should still see your dog after you've provided initial care.

93 Get yourself a good pet first aid manual

There are several on the market and many pet first aid courses will include one. An accurate guide can be handy for treating minor injuries and illnesses at home, and it can also be useful for knowing when it's time to seek professional medical help. Keep it by your first aid kit so you can find it quickly and easily.

94 Have a pet first aid kit at home <u>and</u> in your car

Knowing appropriate first aid is an important first step, but having the tools to properly administer it shouldn't be overlooked. Many companies and stores sell pet first aid kits, or you can put one together yourself. Talk to your veterinarian about recommended supplies or see the list we've put together as a blog post on our website.

95 Program important phone numbers into your cell phone for quick reference while traveling or in the event of an emergency

Having the phone numbers for your veterinarian and for one of the animal poison control hotlines programmed into your phone can save you time, money, and stress. It may well save your pup's life, too. You can find information on recommended pet poison control hotlines on the *Resources* page of our website.

96 Get a good pet health insurance policy

The costs of veterinary care, especially for treatments resulting from emergencies or chronic illnesses, can be quite high. Bills can often run well into the thousands of dollars. These costs will continue to increase as further advances come to veterinary medicine and more pets benefit from seeing veterinary specialists. Having a good insurance policy—particularly for emergencies and illnesses—can give you financial peace of mind. Insurance can also protect you from having

to base important decisions about your pup's medical care solely on finances. For more information on finances in pet emergencies, please see the *Costs of Pet Emergencies* blog post on our website.

Felix, a two-year-old Chihuahua, was attacked by a larger dog one day while playing at the dog park. He suffered bite wounds to his chest and abdominal cavities, requiring extensive surgeries, chest tubes, and prolonged care in the ICU. He recovered fully, though now only goes to the dog parks with separate "small dog" areas. His owners were thankful that they never had to think twice about the significant costs for the life-saving care Felix required—they had signed him up for pet insurance shortly after his first puppy visit to their vet.

Scan this QR code for information and additional resources pertaining to financial preparedness for routine and emergency pet care.

97 Learn how to check your pup's temperature, pulse, and breathing rate

Knowing how to check these three important vital signs in your pup, as well as knowing what is normal for her, can help you determine when there is a problem that might warrant a trip to the vet. Typical "normal ranges" vary based on your pup's size, breed, medical status, and several other factors. What's important is what is normal for *your* pup. Have your veterinarian or one of their technicians show you how to check these vital signs. You don't need to check them on a regular basis, but you should determine what is normal for your pup and check whenever you are concerned. This is information you should learn in any pet first aid class, too.

98 Keep copies of your dog's current medical records on hand

These copies can help you avoid repeated tests in the event that you wind up at another vet's office after hours or while on vacation. Both at home and when you travel, having your pup's records handy can save you time and money. Up-to-date records will also help guard your pup's health and safety by ensuring that any attending veterinarian is aware of the pre-existing conditions or medication allergies she may have. Technology is making this ever-easier—talk to your veterinarian about electronic and online medical records, as well as useful smartphone apps.

99 Know about third-party financing options when faced with unexpected expensive veterinary procedures

If an emergency or illness strikes before you've signed your dog up for insurance, be aware that third-party financing options exist (e.g. CareCredit). Since most vet practices don't do payment plans, these resources can help to soften the initial financial blow of unexpected medical costs. Just be sure to read the fine print and make the required minimum payments or you'll be slapped with a surprisingly high APR. See the *Costs of Pet Emergencies* blog post on our website for more information and links.

100 In poisoning cases, <u>never</u> induce vomiting until you've spoken with a veterinarian

In some cases and with some toxins, causing your dog to vomit is *not* a safe course of action. In these instances, vomiting can actually be more dangerous for your dog than the poison she swallowed. Call your veterinarian, your local animal emergency hospital, or a dedicated animal poison control hotline before taking this step in any poisoning emergency.

101 Know the location of your closest animal emergency hospital, and know how to get there before the need arises

In some emergencies, time can truly be of the essence. Having this information on hand, both at home and when you travel with your pet, can save their life and minimize your stress. Links to find veterinary emergency hospitals throughout North America can be found on the *Resources* page of our website.

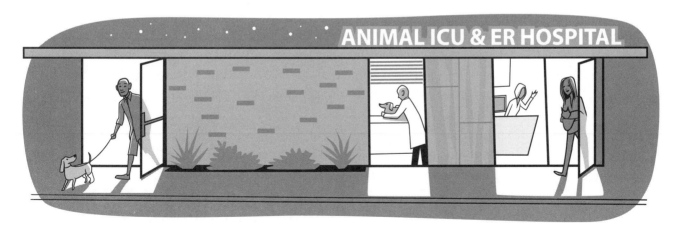

ANIMAL ICU & ER HOSPITAL

Bonus Tip

Scan this QR code to see a cool time-lapse video of another common household hazard that all dog owners should be aware of.

About the Author

Dr. Jason Nicholas, "The Preventive Vet", is an emergency room and general practice veterinarian who spent the early years of his career diagnosing and treating the illnesses and emergencies that he has now helped countless pet owners prevent. True to his professional motto—"Be Aware. Be Prepared. Be Preventive!"—he launched his website, ThePreventiveVet.com, in 2011 to empower pet owners with the information, advice, and resources they need to best protect their pet's health and safety—all from an experienced veterinarian. He is the resident pet expert for the *More Good Day Oregon* show, as well as being a regular contributor to a variety of pet health and safety articles, both in print and online. He lives in Portland, Oregon with his wife, two young daughters, and their wonderful rescue dog, Wendy.